Life in Spite of a
DEATH SENTENCE

© *by Eileen Sammons Tidwell*
from the diary of
John Harlow Sammons
[1944-1994]

Cover Photograph from the collection of
Donna Sammons

For my beloved brother, my hero
John Harlow Sammons   1944-1994

For Donna, the love of his life
And his sons Dennis and Paul

And for All who may face cancer

Opinions and viewpoints are those
of the late John Harlow Sammons
and Eileen Sammons Tidwell
and are not represented to be
anything otherwise.

And In Appreciation:

Our Family and its unlimited ability to love

Our Church Families

Our many friends who encouraged this publication

Prologue

If my brother Johnny had not been such a positive, humorous, upbeat person, I probably would have been even more devastated when he called to tell me he had cancer. But right from the start it was him reassuring me, not the other way around.

He was feeling good and looking great. I witnessed how he looked when he came to Texas from his home in Colorado to visit our mother in 1989. I had called to tell him I didn't think she would last much longer. As it turned out, he arrived only hours after she had died.

The biggest comfort in this double tragedy was that we did not have to try to hide his condition and she never knew her youngest had terminal cancer.

You will find a few helpful sources of information at the end of this story. My brother's experience taught me that it is very important to take a strong pro-active role in our own health.

He had titled his writings "Death Sentence". I have re-titled it to reflect the joy of life he found even while making that journey through the Valley of the Shadow.....--
Eileen Sammons Tidwell

The Diagnosis – a death sentence or a call to arms?

Cancer isn't just another word; it is a sentence... a death sentence straight from Hell.

OK it is a word, but [to victims] it is the most deadly word in the English language. Just telling a man he has CANCER may kill him. It really is a death sentence, complete with all the guilt and sorrow, and it usually produces the same sequence of events and final results.

Does this mean that you will die if Cancer visits you? Not at all! It does mean that we have an incredible fear of this disease. But look at it this way: life is a death sentence yet we don't normally dwell on dying until someone gives us a scenario of how individually we are to die.

When my doctor, in March of 1989, told me that I had prostate cancer, I may have mispronounced "prostate" as "prostrate", but I sure as hell knew what "cancer' meant. It was one of those moments you never forget, come hell, high water or Alzheimer's. I was at work in the art lab; away from my desk when our receptionist told me Doctor R was on line one.

My wife came into the room when she heard the receptionist page me and stared at me, waiting for the decision.

I took the call in the lab with trembling anticipation. "Please God; let me hear the word 'benign'." Surely with others in the same room with me, the Cancer monster would not announce himself with this call.

I had initially been referred to Dr R, a urologist, after a routine physical earlier in the year. He had performed a digital rectal exam and confirmed what the General Practitioner had suspected -- something was wrong in there. He explained that the prostate did not feel normal. When I questioned him, he briefly explained that he thought there might be a tumor, but that prostate problems were extremely rare for someone only forty-four years old. If it was a tumor, it might or might not be malignant. That was about all he would divulge without further tests.

He wanted to do an ultrasound and needle biopsy of the prostate. We set the test up for the following week and I hoped and prayed a little that everything was going to be OK.

No such luck. Malignant.

I gave Donna a thumbs-down sign, put the urologist on hold (probably a thirty five dollar charge to my insurance company) and stumbled back to my office, where upon I found that we needed to meet as soon as his schedule would allow. According to him and other people I had talked with, it might still be in a containable and "curable" stage. The doctor could schedule some tests and give me a reasonable indication of whether we were still in this "cancer abort" window, but he wouldn't know for sure until he had cut me open.

So, the jury was in; the intrusive ultrasound and biopsy had proven that I was guilty of possessing a large malignant tumor within my male reproductive tools. The next step was for the judge (my doctor) to weigh the evidence and determine my sentence. He informed me that it was within my rights to get additional counsel (a second opinion) at any time during the sentencing and appeals process.

I really wasn't clear about the tests. As I understood it, if when they opened me up, or if the tests conclusively showed that it had spread to other regions, there was no reason to remove the prostate. It would be the old line you always hear: "Poor Harlow, they cut into him and he was eaten up with the cancer; there was nothing for them to do but sew him up and let him die".

I hung up, and sobbingly gave Donna the verdict. We hugged each other tightly as we both fell into a state of shock. My partner came in; I told him; more sobbing and my second hug of the long ordeal. Donna and I went home to bed and stayed there, hiding under the covers, trembling and crying for quite some time.

I did not take the news like a man. Not being a man, Donna, thankfully didn't take it like one either.

Finally, we called our good friend Pete, who had lost his wife to breast cancer in 1986. More crying on both ends of the line, but Pete is a doctor and he began the long process of helping us cope with the monster. At the time he told me, "Harlow, there are going to be good days and bad days and you must face them one day at a time. Don't let the bad days take away the good times. "My reaction at the time was, "he's saying I may not get over this thing. Everything is not alright after all". However, as the days and years passed, I grew to appreciate the wealth of wisdom and experience he conveyed with that simple statement.

By the next day I was making one of those little recoveries: Yes, I had CANCER, but I was very young and I wasn't ready to die yet.

I called the Doc and he quickly scheduled a bone scan and a CT scan, and we discussed an immediate (early March) surgery date, if the tests were OK. I mentioned that I had an important business meeting in Billings for late in the month and would it be OK to attend this meeting before the surgery. The kindly doctor informed me that prostate CANCER is slow growing and that three weeks would not make any difference in his ability to save my life. We scheduled the surgery for the Monday before Easter.

For behind-the-times-medical-term collectors like me, a CT (Computed Tomography) scan is often called a "CAT scan". With a name like CAT scan I had always pictured it involving something like the restringing of a tennis racket; I had no idea how it worked, but later learned the CT scan produces sliced photographs of the insides of your key organs, enabling the specialists to see what's happening in the organs.

My doctor had indicated the CT might show any unusual lymph nodes, a sure sign of progression to other sites.

The bone scan is a tiny picture of your skeleton, produced by radioactive isotopes that have been injected into you by specialists dressed in all kinds of lead lined clothing. (I do exaggerate a bit). The particles go to "hot spots" of unusual cell growth and show areas of bone loss giving another expert the opportunity to utilize his interpretive skills to indicate cancerous activities within the skeleton.

One of the first places cancer cells move to once they enter your blood stream is your bones.

I learned that my CT was clear, but that the bone scan showed two areas of concern in the hip. It was possible they were old injuries. Surgery would proceed.

The Surgery and Recovery

I gradually awoke mid-afternoon on Monday before Easter to find Donna and our good friend Lynn waiting. I felt my crotch, found it bandaged and discovered a large tube coming out of my . For the next four weeks this was the focus of my attention. I couldn't move without it hurting. While I had been under the knife Donna and Lynn, a close friend and registered nurse, had discussed the desirability of an oncologist as well as a urologist. Lynn had insisted that we should have seen one before deciding to accept Dr R's prescription for surgery, and that we should still consult with one as soon as possible.

After the surgery, while I was still lost in space, Donna asked Dr. R about a good oncologist. He said he would find one to meet with us.

Maybe I was free of cancer, maybe not; the good doctor just didn't know. Upon opening me up he discovered that the cancer had escaped the "capsule" that encloses the prostate and it had totally consumed one lymph node that sat on the outer side of the capsule; however, the distillate nodes (those close to the prostate) were totally clear. He decided to proceed, but as he was putting me back together he discovered that it had also spread into the neck of my bladder, which required a partial removal of the bladder neck. There was a chance I would fully recover, and there was chance it would return. I chose "fully recover" as my planned option.

A new doctor, Dr F appeared on the scene and proposed that I begin immediate radiation of the bladder/prostate region as an attempt to clean up any remaining cancer cells. Dr R insisted that I wait six weeks to allow healing first.

Six weeks cease fire with cancer, or would it simply spread?

Dr F also introduced a new term to us that controlled my life from then on – PSA - which stands for Prostate Specific Antigen. This is a blood test that measures the level of what is known as a tumor marker, something that only turns up with prostate cancer activity.

Dr. F said my PSA was slightly above normal, and that there was still some activity.

He told us the half life of the antigen would mean that it should still be elevated right after surgery, and I didn't know what to think. So I didn't.

I got out of the hospital on Easter Sunday and we went to lunch with close friends. For the next three weeks I went to work and Donna hauled me around Denver looking at houses, while the catheter in my transported urine to a collection bag and down the side of my leg. Damn, that was so uncomfortable that I still cringe when I think about it.

But time passed and things sort of returned to normal. I began eating food in large quantities, thinking I couldn't die if I ate enough. In June after the radiation was complete, I had another bone scan and the doctor reported the spots had not changed.

Everything was going to be OK! Right? Not quite. After the catheter was removed I discovered that I had severe incontinence and that I was impotent.

Note from Eileen, California Fun:

Johnny had to be in California that spring on business; I flew out to join him. We were very fortunate to have a generous uncle offer us the use of his home while we were there. Uncle was out of town so we shared it only with his dog and his part time household help.

We got out and about, exploring haunts from our childhood visits. We even managed to find our grandmother's old home where she lived when we visited as children. We were ecstatic that it was still there being as a big freeway had been built only two blocks from it. We ate Johnny's wellness diet of beans, vegetables and fruit; we walked and walked and talked and talked and laughed non-stop. We felt good. We laughed and played like children, as indeed we were for that brief few days. We enjoyed that time as we would never enjoy another, just two kids again.

Achieving a Lifetime Goal

Still, as the spring, summer and fall passed, I began to think that I had indeed gotten lucky; that I was going to survive. I resumed work, we traveled and I finally achieved a lifetime goal on October 2, 1989.

I had begun bowling in high school leagues back in 1959 and had continued to bowl in leagues and tournaments. I am a good bowler and in my younger years had planned on a pro career; but not being great enough, I eventually settled for being a Certified Public Accountant. I guess, in retrospect that they were equally unglamorous goals.

At any rate, I had only recently reached the exalted level of a two hundred average bowler and I had never bowled a perfect game.

Well, lo and behold on Monday night, October 2, 1989, while wearing a pad to absorb leakage, it happened.

I had started my second game of the evening with eleven strikes in a row. As I stood up to bowl, a pleasant calmness developed within me. This might be my last chance so don't screw it up I said to myself. The ball rolled along the edge of gutter, and at the last instant, it jumped toward the sacred pocket, scattering pins in all directions. A weight fell off me and I felt like I just floated into the air. It was perhaps the most euphoric feeling I've had.

I still take pride in that accomplishment, feeling that I am probably the only person to ever admit to bowling a "300" in diapers.

I was bowling as well as I ever had in my life in 1989 and in the spring of that year our team had made its annual commitment to bowl in the 1990 American Bowling Congress tournament to be held early 1990 in Reno, NV. I fully intended to be healthy enough to attend, and bowl well in that tourney.

Other positive things happened in the summer and fall of '89 as well. I negotiated a sale of some stock and debentures in my business (along with my partners) which seemed destined to make our publication (*OUTPOST MAGAZINE*) a very successful venture. Additionally Donna and I found really nice home in Denver were able to purchase it; the timing was perfect.

But still: How quickly things change.

In November while driving to Dodge City, KS on business, shoulders and left hip ached badly.

By year's end, we knew IT was back.

1990 – The Roller Coaster Ride

Reflections in 1990: With only a decade left of the 20th Century, it seems there should be more excitement about the approach of the twenty-first century. There should be reflection about the ending of the only century that nearly all of us have ever known. At least it seems that way to me.

I don't know, but I believe that we are obsessed with nightmares about the world today and what it will be like tomorrow. We don't look forward with any excitement and joy; instead we fantasize about our past and how wonderful it was. We cling to images of the past and dread the future. Maybe that is why we seem to be avoiding the impending turn of the century dial.

Certainly in Donna's and my circumstances the future was frightening as 1990 began.

The cancer was real.

Sacrificing some body parts and functions had not satisfied the "demon," so the year began in a veil of tears and fears.

However, the year turned out to be the most exciting "roller coaster ride" we have ever experienced. We sank, we soared, we cried and we roared together as the year slipped along.

By year's end we were back at the "turnstile" and ready to face another spin. How long could the ride last? We didn't ask. We had, at least momentarily, come to accept the current moment in time as the focus of life. It seems in retrospect we were living life at its fullest as the year ended.

Here is what happened in 1990.

A PSA and a bone scan in early January, 1990 confirmed that I had abnormal prostatic growth and metastasis to the bone. The scan showed lesions to the hips, spine, ribs, shoulder blades and skull. Dr R explained that I now definitely had prostatic cancer in my skeleton and its next likely locales would be in the liver and/or lungs.

Wait a minute, if have cancer in my bones, I have bone cancer right? If it goes to the liver or lungs, I have liver or lung cancer, right?

"No," the medical pros told me, "each type of cancer has its own unique set of deviation characteristics." Prostate cancer remains prostate cancer where ever it roams. In a way, that was good news, I only had one type of cancer to worry about.

Actually, the type of cancer at that time was irrelevant to me. The question was, 'How do we get rid of it? What happens now?"

Hormonal therapy. I had a choice of an orchiectomy (castration) or getting monthly shots that would block the manufacture of testosterone by the testicles. What a choice; be a eunuch or be a neo-eunuch.

Actually, it wasn't a hard decision (no pun intended) for me. I had been born with an undescended testicle that had been removed in the early 1970s and I had been frequently warned to watch for testicular cancer.

I was already impotent, incontinent and very much afraid of dying.

Hello castration.

Dr R by this time had developed a high level of respect for Dr. F's knowledge of advanced treatment possibilities, and suggested that I consult with him.

Dr F met with me and explained that prostate cancer is believed to feed on testosterone; elimination of the "food source" would starve the villain.

In addition to the testicles, the adrenal glands produced a substantial supply. He prescribed a three time per day dosage of Flutamide, a medication that blocks the production of testosterone by the adrenal glands. This combined treatment of castration and the use of Flutamide hopefully would produce at least a partial remission of the disease. We would monitor it with the PSA blood tests and a bone scan later in the year.

I add as a reference for other prostate cancer patients: there is a school of thought that insists this medication must be taken every eight hours, not just three times per day (such as breakfast, lunch and dinner), because it is only effective for about 8 hours and the patient should not have periods of exposure.

Neither of the doctors had given me survival statistics for this stage, but I had been informed by both that the chance was small and survival of five years was very unlikely. This limited knowledge was damaging and beneficial at the same time. Fear of the unknown created a sense of doom and despair, but, at the same time, the lack of specific statistics allowed me to retain some hope.

Even though Dr R indicated that the orchiectomy could result in at least a partial remission, he also implied that it was almost certain to return. Not good news.

Telling Our Loved Ones

We now had to tell our sons, Dennis and Paul, and our close friends and relatives that the "miracle" was over, and that there was almost no chance of long term survival.

I remember my youngest son's reaction. He retreated to his room and cried for several hours. Then he shrugged it off as though saying "it's not true, you are my father, you're stronger than any disease and I know you are not going to die." He put his confidence in me and eventually, I began to accept it, learning to face the bad as well as the good with a confidence I never thought was within me.

My sister Eileen's reaction, as she said later on, was like she "had been kicked in the gut." Although we had always been close, this reaction startled me and made me wonder: "Can I really be of that much significance to another?" It may have been perverse, but the emotions my crisis instilled in others eventually created a sense of goodness, beauty and joy within me.

For the moment however, it was back to hiding under bed covers, as fear and shock possessed our bodies and minds. We had initially told our sons about cancer and my chances for survival and all of us had chosen to think I was going to be OK. Now, I had t had to tell them that we were wrong and that I was "probably going to die."

The Spiritual Awakening

As a family, we had never attended any church or placed any emphasis on spirituality and religion. We had inadvertently preached to our sons that good behavior made one good and bad behavior made one bad.

It was hard to believe in God. I didn't really know what He was supposed to be, not having experience with religious training. I can't speak for the rest of my family, but I clung to a belief in the "Golden Rule" and a hybrid form of "Karma" where thoughts and actions affected an all-powerful God's treatment of me. I accepted that He was punishing me for variations from my internal highway of righteousness. With my own unique God, I had a chance to have consequences, such as the Cancers minimized or even pardoned.

Consequently, religion played a changing but major role, in my dance with death.

For most of my life I had professed to be an agnostic, praying to God when something seemed hopeless; usually telling God in my prayers that I would forever believe and behave if he would grant my prayerful request. It seemed natural that I would resort to this behavior again.

But this time was different. For the first time in my life, I gave up my conditions of belief to God and asked only for strength in dealing with my own death.

It came immediately; something internally spoke to me, "Quit dwelling on death and start living like you want to live forever. Maybe the cancer will kill you, but don't just curl up and die from it."

I got out of bed, went back to work and began living again.

We joined an Episcopal Church that was in our neighborhood, because Donna had been an Episcopalian prior to our marriage, and I made a conscious effort to open my mind to the Bible and organized religion.

I was pleasantly surprised to find that Episcopalism, as a whole, seemed to have an attitude of questioning as well as an element of faith. As I sat in church one Sunday, listening to Pastor Sandy Wilson, discuss the concept of the Trinity, I was at last able to accept Jesus.

In 1990, I was finally able to honestly tell my elder Baptist sister Betty that I believed. She had worried about my soul all my life.

More importantly though, I was able to let go of worry and fear about things that were currently out of my control. I could now focus my attention on dealing with problems day by day basis. I did not have to continually face "future" problems anymore; I would deal with them when they got to the present.

Well that's probably enough about "Harlow's great spiritual awakening," let's get back to what happened in 1990.

Cansurmount and Qualife and the Wellness Weekends

Donna and Lynn had their heads together again, discussing support groups and talking to other cancer patients. Cansurmount, a national support organization based in specific hospitals had been contacted, and from there we discovered a different new local group.

Qualife had been founded in 1987 by Dr Paul Hamilton and some of his patients and staff to help cancer patients and their families face the issues and challenges before them. It provided a wide array of support for both patients and family members. As a result of Qualife, we participated in special support groups.

Donna joined a group comprised of family support members that focused on dealing with and helping cancer patients and themselves in facing a new life threatening environment.

I joined a patient support group that was comprised mostly of women with breast cancer. We met weekly and discussed our lives, our fears and hopes, and the lives, fears and hopes of our loved ones.

As the only male in the group, these meetings allowed me to provide a different element of support and encouragement to the ladies of the group. This in turn provided me with a real sense of usefulness and goodness.

But the real benefit of Qualife for me was the Wellness Weekend. I have never been one to join groups or to have much faith in learning from groups, but when Donna enrolled me in this two and one-half day hands-on seminar on life and death, I actually looked forward to meeting other people who were facing the same challenge. Never in my thoughts prior to this week-end did I anticipate what was about to happen.

The meeting was held in the rotunda of an old tuberculosis asylum that was being converted to a Cancer treatment center. The buildings were spread around in a campus-like setting, I remember Canadian Geese wandering the grounds, creating a real sense of peace. As I walked in Friday morning, I was welcomed by smiling energetic faces and the sounds of beautiful, uplifting music. Our first chore was to create name tags so that we could quickly learn each other's names. Mine was unimaginative but it served its purpose. From there things just kept getting better.

I met two fellow prostate cancer patients. Bob Burch, Ed McMahon and I "bonded" as they say and I listened as both of them bragged about their surgeon who was with the University Of Colorado Medical Center.

I was already aware of this doctor's name. He had made national news recently with the results of a "double blind" study of Lupron (the testosterone block) and Flutamide (the adrenal block.) The study indicated that use of these hormonal blockers together increased a patient's life expectancy by eleven months. I had asked my Oncologist, but he had seemed more or less uninterested.

I wondered to myself, should I perhaps talk this physician, but I decided to stay with Dr R and Dr F for the time being.

At any rate, as the week-end progressed we learned about meditation, about breaking through barriers, about nutrition, about trust and, most importantly to me, about "bone pointing."

One of the speakers, Dr J, a clinical psychologist, displayed a carved bone that he had acquired in Central America.

Supposedly, it had once belonged to a "shaman" of some tribal civilization in Central or South America.

According to Dr J, this Shaman would call a tribal meeting whenever someone had committed a serious offense. If serious enough, the Shaman might point the carved bone at the offender in front of the entire tribe.

According to the doctor, the members of the tribe believed so absolutely in the power of the Shaman that the offender would die.

Bone pointing: Could the effects be the same in a society such as ours, when doctors tell their patients that they only have a certain amount of time to live.

You damn right they could. I knew right then, with my weaknesses in the area of suggestion, that I did not need any doctors estimating my remaining time in this body.

On Saturday, we were faced with a challenge, a challenge to push ourselves, to face fear and to try. Could each of us break a piece of plywood with a bare hand?

Yes! I saw a seventy year old woman with arthritic hands break a wooden plank with her bare hands. In fact every one of us accomplished this feat. We all learned to break out of our walls of confinement and to not be afraid of the unknown.

On the final day, the patients and family and support members were divided up, in what seemed random fashion, into two groups. One group was to consist of blind individuals, needing technical and emotional help from a member of the other group.

I was one of the providers and it was my job to help a blind (folded) individual work his/her way through a difficult obstacle course. This course would have been intimidating to nearly anyone with sight, and it sure as heck scared me. My task was to help a fellow human and I had to do it without any verbal communication.

As I walked through the course with the other "helpers," I feared that I would not have the creativity or the strength to be useful. Could I really be of enough help to someone?

Yes, I found out as we conquered the final challenge. I could and I had! This surprising event at the end of perhaps the most meaningful week-end in my life was the perfect climax.

I came home from the weekend feeling more alive I had ever felt in my life. The Wellness Week-end introduced me to a new world of hope and joy. It substantiated my new self confidence, it truly gave meaning to life and gave me a happiness that has been my well spring ever since.

In the days that followed, I took joy in a tremendous sense of beauty and spirituality.

Spring was some time off, but to me it was already here. With true sense of rebirth, I awoke early and took increasingly long leisurely walks, listening to and watching birds, and admiring the neighborhoods and homes that comprise northeast Denver.

I was convinced that a regimen of healthy foods, meditation and exercise would help me stop or slow the onslaught of cancer and provide me with peace and happiness. It did.

The walks became marathon in length and I began to jog much of the way. Excess weight melted from my body and I just kept getting better.

Still Donna and friends of ours insisted that we should be seeking independent opinions on the treatment process.

Second Opinions and More

Our many friends and relatives in Texas insisted that M.D. Hospital was the source of all hope in advanced treatment. A little checking around by my physician got me an 8 AM appointment for a Friday in late February with a renowned oncologist specializing in Prostate Cancer at M.D Anderson.

The only problem was that I was supposed to be in Reno for the ABC Bowling Tournament the day before my appointment.

No problem, my normally penny pinching bride decided. She purchased an additional $800 air fare from Reno to Houston and back to Denver just to get his opinion.

It was a brief encounter. Hormonal therapy was definitely the best therapy at this juncture and anything he could give me would make me much sicker than I currently was. "Go home and wait until you are really sick, then we'll help you."

OK, I decided, we wasted $800 on airfare, but we had the assurance that our care at this time was appropriate. We were on the right track...if a run-a-way train didn't catch us by surprise.

Indeed my life prospects seemed strong. By April of 1990, the dreaded PSA was at absolute zero. No abnormal prostate activity. For the moment I had prostate cancer whipped. Naturally, the results encouraged a continuation of the new life style.

I enrolled in another Wellness Week-end, this one in conjunction with the OUTWARD BOUND organization for the exclusive benefit of Qualife participants.

In June, eight of us along with three director/guides began another weekend of learning about and experiencing life at its fullest. This weekend was conducted outdoors in the central Rocky Mountains near Leadville, CO and was as fulfilling as the initial one. We focused on facing fear and learning about failure. The two weekends taught me things I wish everyone could know.

At the initial weekend we were asked to identify, individually, our greatest fear. As we discussed specific fears we learned that the fear of failure was the source of our specific fears.

The pure fact: If we will not try, we will not succeed. Whether it is breaking boards, rope walking in mountain pines or trying to help another person (or yourself), the only way we are going to really fail is by refusing to try in the first place. Special weekends to learn some basics of life. Rewarding!

The end of June brought us disquieting health news. The PSA results showed a level of 1.0, a rise, but still below the normal or acceptable level, I was told.

Actually this information was incorrect. With the complete removal of the prostate, one's PSA should never be above .02 (the margin of reading error) if there is no malignant activity.

Still I held onto my new sense of peace and continued preparations for a half-marathon run in the mountains west of Denver.

Imagine, here was a forty-six year old man, who had been at least forty pounds overweight for much of his adult life, running in a 13 mile race in the mountains of Denver.

Would I finish it? Of course. The same day? Well, maybe.

Yes, I did, without even changing my diaper! Life was good and God was great.

New Symptoms and New Directions

By this time though, we were becoming aware that all was not OK with the old nemesis, prostate cancer. My stamina was decreasing, and I had a persistent headache that would not go away. Something was not right; l feared a brain tumor.

From visits with my doctor at his laboratory, it was obvious: trouble was coming and he did not have any miracle up his sleeve for me.

It was during this time that I truly began taking a more active role in my medical treatment. Until then, Donna, and my physicians had led the way. Now it was time for me to start leading instead of being led.

We discussed the possibility that the activity was still restricted to the bladder area. I revisited Urologist, for an inside look. I prefer not to go into the process, other than to say that the results showed an all clear in the urinary tract.

The headaches grew in intensity and I returned to see the oncologist. New CT scans and bone scans revealed additional growth in the bones but supposedly no soft tissue tumor activity that would be the cause of the headaches. Good news, no brain tumors...yet.

He suggested a further visit to my primary physician, but I suggested that instead we should get the opinion of a famous Dr C.

He agreed and scheduled a meeting for me supplied the new doctor with necessary medical records and history.

This appointment produced unwanted results for me. The first thing he said, after reviewing my records, was something to the effect of *"I'm sure you know that you will be dead within nine months if you don't get on some treatment program that will impair the cancer. Unfortunately, I don't have anything that will do you any good."* What a great guy! I walk in and he tells me I'm a dead man unless I do something, but he doesn't know what.

Actually though, he did suggest that I contact a urologist at the University of Maryland who was doing some experimentation with a drug called Suramin.

With only six months to live, I didn't dawdle about contacting him. Another opinion came from this guy. According to him, with my PSA only in the single or even double digits, I wasn't sick enough for his protocol.

So it was back to Dr F. I told him what Dr. C had said and that I couldn't get into the Suramin test at the University of Maryland.

Dr. F was preparing to go to a conference of oncologists specializing in Prostate Cancer. He would get the scoop on new stuff.

By early October, I was having visions; actually double vision. And the headaches were continuing. On a recent business trip to Las Vegas the double vision had become intolerable. Probably because with double vision I saw myself losing money at the blackjack tables twice as fast as normal.

Upon returning from Las Vegas I revisited my oncologist.

At his conference he had met the head of prostate cancer research at the National Institute of Health (NIH).

NCI was doing a major study with this "Suramin" stuff and, based upon my condition, was interested in including me in the program. All that had to happen was that I had to contact them, gather up all of my medical records and go visit the National Cancer Institute at the NIH.

Dr F said I seemed to be the type of patient that wanted to try new therapies and have a role in the decision making process and that he thought the Suramin treatment at the NCI could be of benefit to me.

Yes, by golly I was a real take charge guy. It's just that I expected the good doctor to contact NCI for me, gather my records up for me and get me out to Bethesda, MD. By gosh, if he would tell me what to do and then do it for me, I would be a take charge type of patient and let a new doctor make some decisions for me.

Nope, it didn't quite work out that way.

Dr F gave me a Xerox copy of a brief summary of the protocol and eligibility requirements from Dr M and said, "Call him up and see if you qualify."

I did (call) and I did (qualify). At least to fly at my own expense to the National Cancer Institute (NCI) (at the National Institutes of Health) to find out if I qualified for the program itself.

Then if I met the requirements, the NIH would pay for my return trip, and all costs of the protocol, including future air fares and a daily living allowance for meals and lodging.

Suddenly, there was hope on the horizon again. Come December 1, 1990 I would be flying back to the NCI and the NIH, in Bethesda, MD to start a new life as a "white rat."

The Family Reunion and off to National Cancer Institute in Bethesda, MD

With the conclusion of a planned reunion after Thanksgiving, Donna and I were scheduled to hop aboard a United jet to Louisville, KY for the annual RV convention. From there, I had another flight scheduled to deliver me to the NCI, where I was supposed to endure eight weeks of experimental therapy.

I am considerably younger than all of my siblings and we all naturally assumed that I would probably be the last to go. As result, there seemed to be a family groundswell to recreate our cohesiveness in a special get together. Therefore we had organized a family reunion for Thanksgiving 1990 at our home in Denver.

My brother and two sisters, their spouses and my cousin Martha and her husband all promised to share that Thanksgiving. The reunion was the first sign that family love and fellowship were about to make an incredible impact in all of our lives. With the visitation of cancer in me, we were determined to not only provide each other with emotional support, but to also take the time to say and do the things that had often been left unsaid and undone. It was a real "love in."

Our new home in Denver filled with laughter and tears of joy, as we recounted the tales of our youths and fairy tales about our past and our ancestors past. The reunion turned to be a once in a life time experience. We reminisced, joked and laughed and cried. It was truly a weekend of giving thanks for all of us.

Note from Eileen, Thanksgiving Gathering:

My husband Harlan and I, sister Betty with husband Bob, brother Mac with wife Peg plus their granddaughters Leoma and Tanya, and our cousin Martha and her husband Danny came to Denver. What a joyful time for all of us.

As always my little brother was funny and positive. One day while walking together in his neighborhood, he asked me if we were meeting two people or four. Because, he quipped, with double vision he just never knew.

Johnny and I attended Mass at his neighborhood Episcopal Church. That was special beyond words. We had never attended a church service together, and I'd never been to an Episcopalian service. So he guided me through all the kneeling and rising. Appropriate to his liberal beliefs, the minister was a black woman. I loved it. I'd always told him he would make a wonderful Christian if he would just let himself.

Hearing him give Thanks at the big, traditional Thanksgiving Day table in his home was a crowning highlight. I had never heard him pray before. It was sweet, sincere and touching. - Eileen

Bethesda, Complications and Delays

The Louisville convention was also a big success and I cautiously started the sabbatical to Bethesda with hopes that normalcy would soon be returning to our lives.

Unfortunately, it was not to be at that time. My participation in the clinical test was not quite ready to be. Hope fizzled and I faced an immediate return to Denver for critical therapy that was to be conducted there.

I had talked with Dr M and been assured that I would probably be able to start the therapy in Bethesda after completing the treatments in Denver.

In spite of its worldwide fame, the NIH is a warm and comforting campus, near the heart of our nation's Capitol. I was ready, I thought.

On the first Friday of December, I made my first appearance at the 4th floor clinic of Building 10 of the NIH in Bethesda at 9:00 AM, meeting Dr M in person for the first time.

After speaking with me briefly, he explained that Dr. C would be in charge of my assessment and treatment but that he would be overseeing everything. He explained that Suramin was not a new drug, that it had originally been developed to treat Sleeping Sickness in Cattle, and that in the early 1980s he and two other researchers at the NCI had begun clinical trials on its effectiveness in retarding cancer growth, specifically prostate cancer. It had shown solid potential, but had also resulted in some very debilitating side effects, and the clinical tests had been suspended for a period of time.

The most severe side effect had been paralysis in the legs but the affected patients had eventually recovered from that. The trials had been rewritten to minimize these effects and the NCI now had a number of patients on a revised protocol that was resulting in positive responses of indefinite length in about 30% of the patients

You are probably saying to yourself that a 30% chance of benefit doesn't seem very promising, and I confess that I also was a bit disappointed by the statistics.

However, I had already been told by Dr F that existing Chemotherapies offered at best about five percent success results.

Also, Dr M was optimistic that the stuff would work in my case and his enthusiasm certainly encouraged me.

However, when Doctor C went over my medical records, the subject of headaches and double vision raised a flag about the appropriateness of Suramin treatment at that time. He telephoned my oncologist to review things and after the conference, it was obvious that I now had two doctors who did not agree on treatment.

Dr C quickly assessed the symptoms as being caused by malignant growth of the Clivus, a small but important bone between the top of the spine and the skull. This growth could be halted by highly targeted radiation and it would have to be done in Denver before we could start the Suramin.

The NCI insisted that I should get another CT scan and Bone Scan to confirm their assessment, so upon my return, I called Dr F and he scheduled the new scans at the hospital in Denver where all of the testing and surgery had been conducted to date.

These scans confirmed the diagnosis and the reading showed the scans of October had indeed shown the same evidence, but that they had been "misread" at that time.

I met with an unhappy Dr F. who recommended that I forget the NCI and begin one of the chemotherapies that he was familiar with, after the six weeks of radiation.

We discussed options about the sources of radiation therapy and decided to utilize a hospital close to my office and thus less intrusive in my daily activity. (The initial radiation treatments to the bladder in June of 1989 had been done at a hospital closer to our home, but a long way from my office.)

I thought maybe Dr F was uncomfortable about the error in scan interpretation by radiologists at the hospital.

At any rate, it seemed appropriate to find a new oncologist here in Denver to coordinate with the local radiologists to radiate the Clivus, and hopefully stop or retard malignant growth in that area. I had every intention of going back to the NCI upon completion of the radiation therapy to begin the delayed experimental therapy, and it was obvious that an Oncologist other than Dr F would be necessary to work with Dr C at the NCI.

Our friend Lynn came through again with the recommendation of Dr Mc, who was associated with the hospital where the radiation therapy was being conducted.

My initial impression of him was that he was oriented toward breast cancer and not necessarily focused on Prostate Cancer, but that he had a willingness to work with me, with the NCI and if necessary, with Dr C.

As 1990 struggled to the finish line, I was already focusing on the starting line for 1991. Radiation therapy had begun and I was already experiencing relief from the double vision. There was sense of optimism in everything I experienced. I had a new team of doctors and I could blame the former team for some, if not all of my problems.

In 1991, Suramin and the new team at the NCI would enable me to beat or at least control the demon.

The death sentence was on hold.

The Rest of the Story,

FINISHING THE BOOK

NOTE from Eileen –
This is as far as my brother's Cancer Diary could be interpreted. In the chaos of losing him, his computer files were partially deleted, and in trying to convert what he had from Macintosh to PC, the ending paragraphs were lost.

What follows is from my perspective at the time. Within another year he began to weaken, losing some use of his arm and hand and his ability to drive. Again I feared the end might be near. He even said that he didn't think he would make it another month.

TNT – Extreme and Experimental

And yet another miracle came . . . another of the many that had already kept him alive and going beyond the original prognosis. Johnny in his proactive search for help, found an experimental -- very experimental -- cancer treatment going on in California.

Called TNT, it involved radioactive isotopes inserted into the bloodstream and programmed to seek out dead tissue. A following isotope zeroed in on the first and zapped cancer tumors. Only a healthy heart could have survived this treatment, because a heart attack leaves dead heart tissue, and that would have attracted the radiation. Johnny was the youngest and in best general health of the volunteers. I think only four were done about that time frame.

During his stay in California for those treatments, he stayed in the homes of first our cousin Martha, and then our Aunt and Uncle, Betty and Ford Sammons. He had been too young when I used to visit with them on the family trips to California, so he had never had the opportunity to really know them. It was a wonderful bonding experience for the three of them.

The improvement in Johnny's health was startling. His arm regained function. He got stronger. He gained back much-needed weight. He resumed his work.

May 1, 1993, I attended Johnny's 49th birthday party at his and Donna's home in Denver. Donna had sent out invitations to "He's Not Dead Yet Birthday Party." That set the tone for the happy time we had together.

The cherry blossoms in Denver reflected the rosy, happy atmosphere of the time there. He was obviously not as strong as when I last saw him, but he was still able to get out and about. We went gambling in Central City, famous for the "Face on the Bar Room Floor. He took me to visit his favorite bookstore, where we spent hours among books, comfortable furniture and interesting people.

On his birthday about 20 people showed up to honor him. Donna had decided on a 'salads' meal, and there were more kinds of wonderful dishes than I could even imagine. All of it healthy stuff! Johnny was still able to get out and go walking so we did a good bit of that too.

But from that point the decline in Johnny's health was steady, although fairly slow. He finally had to step down from his position in his company and became bedfast.

My daughter Danni, a nurse, spent a few weeks with him while Donna was traveling on business. After that he had home health care.

FIVE YEARS AFTER DIAGNOSIS - May 1994 – But he did make it to his 50th birthday, May 1, 1994. He died later that month.

John Harlow Sammons' Memorial Service was held in Idaho Springs, CO., the town where he had been a civic leader. The service drew townspeople, family, friends, acquaintances and people whose lives had been touched during his fight with cancer, some coming from Bethesda, MD.

It was a joyful celebration of life, with people standing to individually eulogize him, sharing memories and his effects on their lives. It was the most inspirational funeral or memorial I have ever attended.

Although he never was able to finish his book about the experience, he did help researchers to develop innovative new treatments, and I am comforted to think that every surviving prostate cancer patient is part of my brother's legacy.

And one big lesson that his story emphasizes is that we must always be actively involved in anything concerning our health. We must be our own best advocates.

John Harlow Sammons: a hero.

– Eileen Tidwell 2009

RESOURCES:

Below is information specific to prostate cancer that I find helpful; there are many others of course. I've tried to be accurate, but please just use these as a guide, not as written in granite sources. Internet links often change and become unavailable.

If you or your loved one has cancer, do your research and be your OWN BEST ADVOCATE.

- *http://www.cancer.gov/cancertopics/pdq/treatment/prostate/patient*
- *http://www.mdanderson.org/?gclid=CMOczcbA-ZwCFado5QodfgOTbA*
- *http://www.cancerresearch.org/resources/what-to-do-if-prostate-cancer-strikes.html*
- *http://www.prostate-cancer.com/*

Stages of Prostate Cancer

http://www.prostate-cancer.com/prostate-cancer-treatment-overview/overview-staging.html

http://www.prostate-cancer.com/prostate-cancer-glossary/stage-T2.html

The American Cancer Society, 1·800·ACS·2345

National Institutes of Health (NIH)

9000 Rockville Pike,

Bethesda, Maryland 20892

800-4-CANCER

CanSurmount:

http://www.stjohnwilderness.org/cansurmount.htm

NOTES:

www.ingramcontent.com/pod-product-compliance
Lightning Source LLC
Chambersburg PA
CBHW070243290526
45789CB00004B/1736